# THE FOOD OF ANGELS

by Dr. Carl K. Barniak

**Barniak Publications**
424 S. Kentucky Ave.
Evansville, IN 47714

Published October 1984 (First Printing)
Printed in the United States of America
ISBN 0-961-38030-6

THE FOOD OF ANGELS is available at quantity discounts with bulk purchase. For information, please write to: Barniak Publications, 424 S. Kentucky Ave., Evansville, IN 47714.

# DEDICATION

**To my family and our Saviour,**
**let the world know, I love you.**

**Dear friend, I pray that you may enjoy good health and that all may go well with you, even as your soul is getting along well. (3 John 2)**

**ACKNOWLEDGEMENT**

As a human with all the physical and intellectual frailities that are typically found to surround such, I humbly recognize those that have carried me past my weaknesses with direction and inspiration. These are the ones that truly deserve whatever good is to be garnished from this project, I being but a pen in the hands of those who are truly wiser. Let their presence be acknowledged.

By our mere being we reflect the will of our God, and each thought passing through our consciousness is realized only through the love of our Creator. Let this work, and all that I do, honestly reflect His will, understanding that without His constant presence nothing would be possible.

I recognize the unfailing support of our mediator, Jesus Christ. Every prayer received an answer, every mental lag a moment of inspiration. Comfortingly, He was always there.

All projects begin, and are sustained, by a desire. Without such internal drive, no inertia is overcome, no conclusion is reached. This all began as but a curiosity, it lead to a book and a desire to know and live God's will. It was the Holy Spirit that planted the seed and furnished the water as needed.

To all, I am grateful. May you be pleased with this work.

# TABLE OF CONTENTS

> **Listen, listen to me, and eat what is good, and your soul will delight in the richest of fare. (Isaiah 55:2)**

## THE LESSON OF THE QUAIL

We are the victims of history, and history does repeat itself. We succumb to the same inappropriate choices that plagued our forefathers, while they repeated the pattern of their fathers. In the areas of real importance, mankind does not learn from its foolishness. Perhaps it is vanity, perhaps it is a feeling that we uniquely are different and that it is the masses, and not I, that must beware. But we are in the midst of history, and the lesson of the quail is again repeating itself. We read:

> **The rabble with them began to crave other food, and again the Israelites started wailing and said, "If only we had meat to eat! We remember the fish we ate in Egypt at no cost—also the cucumbers, melons, leeks, onions and garlic. But now we have lost our appetite; we never see anything but this manna!" (Numbers 11:4-6)**

With infinite wisdom, God directs our actions. He encouraged Moses and his Israelite followers to eat manna in their journey through the desert from Egypt, and not meat, for good reason. The Psalmist tells us:

> **Therefore the Lord heard this, and was wroth: so a fire was kindled against Jacob, and anger also came up against Israel; Because they believed not in God, and trusted not in his salvation: Though he had commanded the clouds from above, and opened the doors of heaven, And had rained down manna upon them to eat, and had given them of the corn of heaven. Man did eat angels' food: (Psalm 78:21-25 KJV)**

God knew that to eat anything but manna, at that time, would lead to ill-health. But man has free-will; when the Israelites pleaded for meat, God gave them quail. Disease, as foretold, would appear among those who ate:

> **Now a wind went out from the Lord and drove quail in from the sea. It brought them down all around the camp to about three feet above the ground, as far as a day's walk in any direction. All that day and night and all the next day the people went out and gathered quail. No one gathered less than ten homers. Then they spread them out all around the camp. But while the meat was still between their teeth and before it could be consumed, the anger of the Lord burned against the people, and he struck them with a severe plague. Therefore the place was named Kibroth Hattaavah, because there they buried the people who had craved other food. (Numbers 11:31-34)**

It is all here within one short story: God's desire for man's good health, the disobedience of man for temporal pleasure, the suffering by man of foretold consequences. The issue here is nutrition, but the theme could be any. The food of angels is not meat, the path to good health is not to be determined by man. God has laid out the plan. Not unlike the ancient Israelites, the choice is now ours.

## INTRODUCTION

From the point of view of one relatively well educated in the biological sciences, and with a practical background in a healing art, I note a tremendous volume of opposing literature on the subject of how to obtain and maintain good health. If modern man is truly learning sciences at the universities, then why the ever-changing, contradictory mass of information on this subject? Why does there remain so much room for divergent opinion on how to get well? After centuries of study and research, why is mankind in such poor physical health, and continuing to spiral downward? Perhaps, the answers to these most important questions are not to be found in the classroom or laboratory, but lie somewhere else.

It strikes my interest that so many people can study the Bible, and so few actually gather more than a handful of Scriptures as proof of their exhausting efforts. If the Bible's guidelines for spiritual fulfillment are valid and meaningful, then why not search-out the remainder of this useful book for direction in other aspects of life? With this idea in mind, I undertook the task of researching the Scriptures for answers to the health concerns of my patients and myself.

I claim not to be an expert in theology, but then again, the experts told Columbus the world was flat. I do claim an ability to learn that which is understandable, and the Bible is understandable. Though not all of the Bible's message is clear, its story is certain to be brought into sharper focus, in time, as God so intended.

An important theme does run through the Bible, being perhaps the best kept secret in the Christian community. Just like God has a plan for all aspects of our lives, God has a plan for our health. To understand and gain from the wisdom of a book, we must first identify exactly that which we want to learn. I sought answers to questions of nutrition, and I was not disappointed by God's response through the word of the Bible. I present my findings to the reader in as clear, concise, and interesting a format as I find possible. Perhaps cleverly, I have ordered my findings into "The Nutritional Commandments of God." Deliberately, I have forced myself to interject as little narrative as possible; enough to maintain a certain flow between Scriptures and provide insight where it is needed, but still backstage to the inherent wisdom of the Bible.

As the well-meaning preacher told his congregation, "Believe not, without question, that which I say, but fail not to believe every word of the Bible." For like the preacher and other erring humans, I, too, make mistakes. Here, with absolute sincerity and singleness of purpose, I have gathered Scriptures. Let you, the reader, assist with the commentary as the logic of God's nutritional message is unraveled before you.

**" 'Go to this people and say, "You will be ever hearing but never understanding; you will be ever seeing but never perceiving." For this people's heart has become calloused; they hardly hear with their ears, and they have closed their eyes. Otherwise they might see with their eyes, hear with their ears, understand with their hearts and turn and I would heal them.' " (Acts 28:26,27)**

## PREMISES

The Bible, and this book, are based upon a number of premises:

1. The Bible is an inspired writing which is the word of God:

**All Scripture is God-breathed and is useful for teaching, rebuking, correcting and training in righteousness, so that the man of God may be thoroughly equipped for every good work. (2 Timothy 3:16,17)**

2. The Bible, being the word of God, is Truth and is meant to be accepted in totality:

**Sanctify them by the truth; your word is truth. (John 17:17)**

**. . . for it is written, "Cursed is everyone who does not continue to do everything written in the Book of the Law." (Galatians 3:10)**

**I warn everyone who hears the words of the prophecy of this book: If anyone adds anything to them, God will add to him the plagues described in this book. And if anyone takes words away from this book of prophecy, God will take away from him his share in the tree of life and in the holy city, which are described in this book. (Revelation 22:18,19)**

**I tell you the truth, until heaven and earth disappear, not the smallest letter, not the least stroke of a pen, will by any means disappear from the Law until everything is accomplished. (Matthew 5:18)**

**Do not add to what I command you and do not subtract from it, but keep the commands of the Lord your God that I give you. (Deuteronomy 4:2)**

**Be strong and very courageous. Be careful to obey all the law my servant Moses gave you; do not turn from it to the right or to the left, that you may be successful wherever you go. (Joshua 1:7)**

3. The Bible, being Truth, is valid for all times:

**"I the Lord do not change. So you, O descendants of Jacob, are not destroyed. Ever since the time of your forefathers you have turned away from my decrees and have not kept them. Return to me, and I will return to you," says the Lord Almighty. (Malachi 3:6,7)**

**"The grass withers and the flowers fall, but the word of our God stands forever." (Isaiah 40:8)**

**Love the Lord your God and keep his requirements, his decrees, his laws and his commands always. (Deuteronomy 11:1)**

**Your word, O Lord, is eternal; it stands firm in the heavens. (Psalm 119:89)**

4. The Bible, being Truth, is valid for all people:

   **Then I saw another angel flying in midair, and he had the eternal gospel to proclaim to those who live on the earth—to every nation, tribe, language, and people. (Revelation 14:6)**

5. Man is an inseparable totality of Spirit, Mind, and Body. The fulfillment of one aspect of man cannot be accomplished without affecting the other parts. The Bible presents guidelines for the enlightenment of all aspects of man:

   **May God himself, the God of peace, sanctify you through and through. May your whole spirit, soul and body be kept blameless at the coming of our Lord Jesus Christ. (1 Thessalonians 5:23)**

6. Finally, the Bible is plainly written and meant to be easily understood by all. It was not meant to be so elusive in its concepts and meanings that only a privileged few Biblical scholars could translate, understand, and gain from its inherent wisdom:

   **The wrath of God is being revealed from heaven against all the godlessness and wickedness of men who suppress the truth by their wickedness, since what may be known about God is plain to them, because God has made it plain to them. For since the creation of the world God's invisible qualities—his eternal power and divine nature—have been clearly seen, being understood from what has been made, so that men are without excuse. (Romans 1:18-20)**

   The Bible's message may be elusive, though, if not earnestly sought after. It is not cast down upon the resisting souls of those entrenched in worldly, not spiritual, matters:

   **The man without the Spirit does not accept the things that come from the Spirit of God, for they are foolishness to him, and he cannot understand them, because they are spiritually discerned. (1 Corinthians 2:14)**

**Your word is a lamp to my feet and a light for my path. (Psalm 119:105)**

## IN SEARCH OF TRUTH

In life, it is so important that one finds Truth. That body of knowledge presented to us by the scientist is not Truth, for science is ever-changing, while Truth does not change. Truth is steadfast against time and critics. It is that unwavering instruction upon which a person, and a society, can build a productive future.

Grecian philosophers through modern scientists have labored unsuccessfully in an effort to find Truth. Before declaring that Truth can not be found, let us look one final place. Let us look to the Bible, the word of God, which has been with us all along.

Reading through the Bible, we find that the Bible itself claims to hold Truth:

**. . . but first I will tell you what is written in the Book of Truth. (Daniel 10:21)**

This would appear logical only if its individual writers, in turn, could be said to possess Truth. God, the obvious mainstay of the Bible, is himself called the God of Truth:

**Into your hands I commit my spirit; redeem me, O Lord, the God of truth. (Psalm 31:5)**

**Whoever invokes a blessing in the land will do so by the God of Truth; he who takes an oath in the land will swear by the God of truth. (Isaiah 65:16)**

Jesus declared that He, too, is Truth.

> **Jesus answered, "I am the way and the truth and the life. No one comes to the Father except through me." (John 14:6)**

Prophets like Elijah, as spokesmen of God, spoke Truth:

> **Then the woman said to Elijah, "Now I know that you are a man of God and that the word of the Lord from your mouth is the truth." (1 Kings 17:24)**

Paul, an apostle, noted in his writings that he too spoke Truth:

> **And for this purpose I was appointed a herald and an apostle—I am telling the truth, I am not lying—and a teacher of the true faith to the Gentiles. (1 Timothy 2:7)**
>
> **As surely as the truth of Christ is in me, nobody in the regions of Achaia will stop this boasting of mine. (2 Corinthians 11:10)**

We should feel confident in accepting the Bible and its inspired writers as a source of Truth. Fortunately for us easily confused humans, God has ordered those Truths most important for daily use into commands, laws, and decrees. These laws are Truths:

> **I have chosen the way of truth; I have set my heart on your laws. (Psalm 119:30)**
>
> **Your righteousness is everlasting and your law is true. (Psalm 119:142)**

Like all Truths, their essence will not change with time:

> **It is easier for heaven and earth to disappear than for the least stroke of a pen to drop out of the Law. (Luke 16:17)**

Man is God's most intelligent creation on Earth. We should reflect that intelligence by letting Truth, not bias or guess, direct our daily actions. Let us refer to those same Truths for proper guidance in our choice of foods for nourishment.

**Anyone who breaks one of the least of these commandments and teaches others to do the same will be called least in the kingdom of heaven, but whoever practices and teaches these commands will be called great in the kingdom of heaven. (Matthew 5:19)**

## A NEW WAY OF THINKING

Perhaps a reason for mankind's failure to determine the keys to superior health lies in the manner of his approach. Classically, the scientific method of reasoning is utilized to discern life's mysteries. A series of isolated facts are taken into account, some common thread is found, and a conclusion is drawn from their conglomerate presence.

In good scientific style, the researcher avoids forming any early conclusions so as not to influence his final verdict. To decide, for example, whether to eat, or not to eat pork, the scientist would consider all available information and draw a logical conclusion upon the data present.

Inherent within the system are certain significant shortcomings:

1. Despite an attempt at precision, original research is often filled with flaws in technique, thus producing faulty end results. To use these erroneous results to derive further conclusions is the basis of an unsound foundation.
2. The scientific conclusion is often formed without access to all, or the best, available information. The scientific truths by which we live change on a daily basis as the bits of isolated information expand and so force an alteration in previously accepted principles. Pork, for example, may seem permissable as food until studies indicate the presence of transmittable parasites within the swine, and thus change one's conclusion concerning its acceptability as food. At any point in time, one will never know if all appropriate data has been collected, thus an ever-changing foundation upon which we base our lifestyle.

Nutritionists have, in most part, relied solely upon the scientific manner of research for direction. Health-care has been fickle as science sways between extremes, with no perceptible hope for the finding of rock-hard Truths at any point in the future.

The revealed manner of thinking is vastly superior, for it begins with the answer and works its way backward in an attempt to show its validity. It streamlines research, for it conveniently disregards all findings which seem to be disproving the known Truth's validity. The researcher works with the hindsight of knowing the end result before collecting the first data. Unfortunately, this advantage rarely is placed in front of the scientist. Without the supposed convenience of being born with life's Truths, man has sought knowledge through the scientific method, recognizing its many limitations, and enduring the hardships posed by such a technique.

Only the Creator of the Universe can know life's Truths. Man can guess and, simply by playing the percentage game, occasionally stumble upon the answers. But what an irritating manner of passing through existence. When God has already given us a share of life's answers, found within the Bible, why waste another moment in searching elsewhere, or another thought in a grasp for the final word? Why resist the convenience of having life's answers neatly given to us by the Creator of life itself?

Let science take a new approach. Let us employ the theologians to first seek out the Bible for its Truths, then let us employ the scientist to explain why it is so.

If the Bible so states that we should not eat pork, let us not, in our vanity, believe that God is wrong and that we know better. Rather, for the sake of brevity and in the name of faith, we should accept the printed word of our Creator, and enjoy the rewards of our good servitude.

**My son, pay attention to what I say; listen closely to my words. Do not let them out of your sight, keep them within your heart; for they are life to those who find them and health to a man's whole body. (Proverbs 4:20-22)**

## NOT JUST A SPIRITUAL WORK

The Bible is not just a spiritual work, for its message in the area of health is strong and clear. Follow its nutritional guidelines and expect good health, or deny the message and suffer foretold consequences:

**"If you listen carefully to the voice of the Lord your God and do what is right in his eyes, if you pay attention to his commands and keep all his decrees, I will not bring on you any of the diseases I brought on the Egyptians, for I am the Lord who heals you." (Exodus 15:26)**

**However, if you do not obey the Lord your God and do not carefully follow all his commands and decrees I am giving you today, all these curses will come upon you and overtake you: (Deuteronomy 28:15)**

Harsh and strange illnesses have always been among men. As science is able to solve each major disease, another of equal magnitude soon appears. This God has promised. Until mankind pays heed to God's health message, physical misery will live among us:

> **The Lord will plague you with diseases until he has destroyed you from the land you are entering to possess. (Deuteronomy 28:21)**
>
> **The Lord will strike you with wasting disease, with fever and inflammation, with scorching heat and drought, with blight and mildew, which will plague you until you perish. (Deuteronomy 28:22)**
>
> **If you do not carefully follow all the words of this law, which are written in this book, and do not revere this glorious and awesome name—the Lord your God—the Lord will send fearful plagues on you and your descendants, harsh and prolonged disasters, and severe and lingering illnesses. He will bring upon you all the diseases of Egypt that you dreaded, and they will cling to you. The Lord will also bring on you every kind of sickness and disaster not recorded in this Book of the Law until you are destroyed. (Deuteronomy 28:58-61)**

Those who have sought their spiritual salvation from the wisdom of the Bible would also be wise to seek out that same author for salvation from ill-health. For one who can promise eternal life for His followers can surely provide a plan of physical vitality for our short earthly stay.

**Because I love your commands more than gold, more than pure gold, and because I consider all your precepts right, I hate every wrong path. (Psalm 119:127,128)**

**Gold there is, and rubies in abundance, but lips that speak knowledge are a rare jewel. (Proverbs 20:15)**

## WHY HAVE WE BEEN GIVEN THE LAWS?

Life, as we all know, often can be both difficult and confusing. The problems that confront us each day demand a solution. A satisfying, fruitful existence is the worthwhile reward for those that consistently provide proper answers to their problems. The Christian, fortunately, has been given a working reference manual for dealing with this constant strife.

The Bible is an act of love by God to assist in life's daily struggle, for those that choose to be His followers:

**I will instruct you and teach you in the way you should go; I will counsel you and watch over you. (Psalm 32:8)**

Apostle Paul notes that the laws reflect God's will and provide us with instruction:

> **if you know his will and approve of what is superior because you are instructed by the law; (Romans 2:18)**

The guidelines for a suitable existence have been neatly ordered into decrees, laws, commands, and requirements. Their difference to us is insignificant, for they are all useful and demand our total respect and compliance:

> **Love the Lord your God and keep his requirements, his decrees, his laws and his commands always. (Deuteronomy 11:1)**

> **He commanded Judah to seek the Lord, the God of their fathers, and to obey his laws and commands. (2 Chronicles 14:4)**

The law of God is good and is not a burden. It is the fence along the pathway of life, providing a tangible border from the harm which besets those who stray off the marked road:

> **My son, do not despise the Lord's discipline and do not resent his rebuke, because the Lord disciplines those he loves, as a father the son he delights in. (Proverbs 3:11,12)**

The laws provide us with a clearer understanding of right and wrong, and they allow us to develop as God desires. In his letter to the Christians of Rome, Paul discussed why we have been given the law:

> **What shall we say, then? Is the law sin? Certainly not! Indeed I would not have known what sin was except through the law. For I would not have known what it was to covet if the law had not said, "Do not covet." (Romans 7:7)**

It is promised that we will prosper when we follow the law, that we will enjoy good health and longevity, and that the law will provide us a basis for solving our daily problems. Are these wishes at all unlike what any good father would want for his children?

**In everything that he undertook in the service of God's temple and in obedience to the law and the commands, he sought his God and worked wholeheartedly. And so he prospered. (2 Chronicles 31:21)**

**Observe therefore all the commands I am giving you today, so that you may have the strength to go in and take over the land that you are crossing the Jordan to possess, and so that you may live long in the land that the Lord swore to your forefathers to give to them and their descendants, a land flowing with milk and honey. (Deuteronomy 11:8,9)**

**Have I not written thirty sayings for you, sayings of counsel and knowledge, teaching you true and reliable words, so that you can give sound answers to him who sent you? (Proverbs 22:20,21)**

**Worship the Lord your God, and his blessing will be on your food and water. I will take away sickness from among you, and none will miscarry or be barren in your land. I will give you a full life span. (Exodus 23:25,26)**

**Enter through the narrow gate. For wide is the gate and broad is the road that leads to destruction, and many enter through it. But small is the gate and narrow the road that leads to life, and only a few find it. (Matthew 7:13,14)**

## THE LAW AFTER CHRIST

The presence of this book and the raising of the issue of nutritional commandments challenges the lifestyle of many Christians and, understandingly, provokes their criticism. This criticism has focussed upon two particular themes:

1. Salvation can be obtained through faith alone, and
2. With the crucifixion of Christ all Old Testament directives are nullified and, therefore, lack pertinence to modern man.

Both noted themes are invalid for lack of supportive Biblical Scripture, and will be addressed separately.

The issue of salvation through faith alone is clearly addressed in the writing of James:

> **What good is it, my brothers, if a man claims to have faith but has no deeds? Can such faith save him? (James 2:14)**
>
> **In the same way, faith by itself, if it is not accompanied by action, is dead. (James 2:17)**
>
> **You see that a person is justified by what he does and not by faith alone. (James 2:24)**

Christ, by thought, word, and action, kept the law of His Father:

> **"Not everyone who says to me, 'Lord, Lord,' will enter the kingdom of heaven, but only he who does the will of my Father who is in heaven." (Matthew 7:21)**
>
> **For it is not those who hear the law who are righteous in God's sight, but it is those who obey the law who will be declared righteous. (Romans 2:13)**
>
> **And I saw the dead, great and small, standing before the throne, and books were opened. Another book was opened, which is the book of life. The dead were judged according to what they had done as recorded in the books. (Revelation 20:12)**

The subject of faith without good deeds was of much concern to the early Christians. The Apostle John discussed the issue:

> **The man who says, "I know him," but does not do what he commands is a liar, and the truth is not in him. But if anyone obeys his word, God's love is truly made complete in him. This is how we know we are in him: Whoever claims to live in him must walk as Jesus did. (1 John 2:4-6)**

To challenge the need for good deeds is to challenge the essence of the law. Paul summarized his feelings on the subject:

> **Do we, then, nullify the law by this faith? Not at all! Rather, we uphold the law. (Romans 3:31)**

Good Christians accept the Ten Commandments from Moses in the Old Testament without hesitation, and doubtlessly feel that these directives are still binding despite the crucifixion of Christ. With the same logic, why then are not all other guidelines of faith, morality, social behaviour, health, and nutrition, given by God before the death of Christ, sound and still binding?

Long before the time of Moses, Adam and Eve were presented with commands from God. Abraham was later also given a set of commandments:

> **"I will make your descendants as numerous as the stars in the sky and will give them all these lands, and through your offspring all nations on earth will be blessed, because Abraham obeyed me and kept my requirements, my commands, my decrees and my laws." (Genesis 26:4,5)**

The Old Testament presents the early history of mankind, the commandments of God, and the prophecies of a coming Saviour. The New Testament describes the fulfillment of these prophecies through the life of Christ, and clarification of God's earlier directives. Christ's purpose was in no way to contradict the message of His Father, rather, He said:

> **"Do not think that I have come to abolish the Law or the Prophets; I have not come to abolish them but to fulfill them." (Matthew 5:17)**

In the lesson of the rich young man (Mark 10:17-31), Christ was asked, "What must I do to inherit eternal life?" Christ responded by saying that the commandments of God, found in the Old Testament, must be followed:

> **You know the commandments: 'Do not murder, . . .' (Mark 10:19)**

Some contend that faith alone is sufficient, that the law was nullified with Christ's resurrection. This is wrong! Christ himself was born under the law and also followed these directives. Redemption is promised to only those who observe the law:

> **But when the time had fully come, God sent his Son, born of a woman, born under law, to redeem those under law, that we might receive the full rights of sons. (Galatians 4:4,5)**

As Christ obeyed the commandments of His Father, we are in-turn told by Christ to follow the law:

> **"If you love me, you will obey what I command." (John 14:15)**
>
> **"If you obey my commands, you will remain in my love, just as I have obeyed my Father's commands and remain in his love." (John 15:10)**
>
> **Jesus replied, "If anyone loves me, he will obey my teaching. My Father will love him, and we will come to him and make our home with him. He who does not love me will not obey my teaching. These words you hear are not my own; they belong to the Father who sent me." (John 14:23,24)**

The true disciples, according to Jesus, are those that follow His teachings, which focussed upon the law:

> **To the Jews who had believed him, Jesus said, "If you hold to my teaching, you are really my disciples. Then you will know the truth, and the truth will set you free." (John 8:31,32)**

The inspired David also stated:

> **I will walk about in freedom, for I have sought out your precepts. (Psalm 119:45)**

The theme is again repeated:

> **"To do your will, O my God, is my desire; your law is within my heart." (Psalm 40:8)**

Simply, God is saying that one *must* prove his faith by following *all* the commandments. Unfortunately, many choose to follow only those commandments which are convenient, while ignoring others under the premise of their being irrelevant:

> **For the time will come when men will not put up with sound doctrine. Instead, to suit their own desires, they will gather around them a great number of teachers to say what their itching ears want to hear. They will turn their ears away from the truth and turn aside to myths. (2 Timothy 4:3,4)**

Looking at mankind's history through the foresight of the Book of Revelation, it is stated:

> **Blessed are they that do his commandments, that they may have right to the tree of life, and may enter in through the gates into the city. (Revelation 22:14 KJV)**

We are also wisely told:

> **This is what the Lord says: "Stand at the crossroads and look; ask for the ancient paths, ask where the good way is, and walk in it, and you will find rest for your souls. But you said, 'We will not walk in it.' " (Jeremiah 6:16)**

> **Hear, O earth: I am bringing disaster on this people, the fruit of their schemes, because they have not listened to my words and have rejected my law. (Jeremiah 6:19)**

> **But the man who looks intently into the perfect law that gives freedom, and continues to do this, not forgetting what he has heard, but doing it—he will be blessed in what he does. (James 1:25)**

The Psalmist has neatly tied together for us the themes of truth, love, law, and eternity:

> **Hear my voice in accordance with your love; renew my life, O Lord, according to your laws. Those who devise wicked schemes are near, but they are far from your law. Yet you are near, O Lord, and all your commands are true. Long ago I learned from your statutes that you established them to last forever. (Psalm 119:149-152)**

**Do not be wise in your own eyes; fear the Lord and shun evil. This will bring health to your body and nourishment to your bones. (Proverbs 3:7,8)**

## DISOBEYING THE LAW IS SIN!

To accept that God has provided guidelines for a superior dietary plan, and that the pursuit of this recommended pattern of eating will lead to a healthier body or personal temple, is good. An important question arises with acceptance of these nutritional directives. Is it a sin NOT to follow the dietary commands passed down to us through the Bible?

As in all important issues, we should develop our logic around the sound basis of Scripture.

The Bible defines sin as a transgression of the law:

**Everyone who sins breaks the law; in fact, sin is lawlessness. (1 John 3:4)**

Sin comes from doing that which is wrong according to the law, or failing to do that which is right. Just like in present society, one may be declared guilty by an act of commission (committing a crime), or by an act of omission (being an accomplice to the crime) by failing to prevent an injustice:

> **All wrongdoing is sin, . . . (1 John 5:17)**
>
> **Anyone, then, who knows the good he ought to do and doesn't do it, sins. (James 4:17)**

Interestingly, those who have not heard the law, yet live in the way the law describes, shall be considered righteous:

> **All who sin apart from the law will also perish apart from the law, all who sin under the law will be judged by the law. For it is not those who hear the law who are righteous in God's sight, but it is those who obey the law who will be declared righteous. (Indeed, when Gentiles, who do not have the law, do by nature things required by the law, they are a law for themselves, even though they do not have the law, since they show that the requirements of the law are written on their hearts, their consciences also bearing witness, and their thoughts now accusing, now even defending them.) (Romans 2:12-15)**

The nutritional commandments are one part of the law of God. The law in total is absolute and inflexible; to break one part of the law is to sin against all of the law:

> **For whoever keeps the whole law and yet stumbles at just one point is guilty of breaking all of it. (James 2:10)**

Fortunate are we all that God's good grace extends down upon all His free-willed sinful people:

> **Blessed is he whose transgressions are forgiven, whose sins are covered. Blessed is the man whose sin the Lord does not count against him and in whose spirit is no deceit. (Psalm 32:1,2)**

**"Why do you ask me about what is good?" Jesus replied. "There is only One who is good. If you want to enter life, obey the commandments." (Matthew 19:17)**

## First Nutritional Commandment
## THOU SHALL PREFER FRUITS, VEGETABLES, NUTS, GRAINS, AND SEEDS

By design, Adam and Eve were meant to enjoy perfect health in Eden. Their food supply was endless, easily accessible, and simple in preparation. There was no death, no need for the slaughter of animals for food. Perfect health was theirs simply by eating the vegetation that God had provided:

**Then God said, "Let the land produce vegetation: seed-bearing plants and trees on the land that bear fruit with seed in it, according to their various kinds." And it was so. The land produced vegetation: plants bearing seed according to their kinds and trees bearing fruit with seed in it and according to their kinds. And God saw that it was good. (Genesis 1:11,12)**

**Then God said, "I give you every seed-bearing plant on the face of the whole earth and every tree that has fruit with seed in it. They will be yours for food." (Genesis 1:29)**

> **". . . everything that has the breath of life in it—I give every green plant for food." (Genesis 1:30)**
>
> **And the Lord God made all kinds of trees grow out of the ground—trees that were pleasing to the eye and good for food. (Genesis 2:9)**

Appetite and curiosity took control of reason. Unable to control their more basic emotions, Adam and Eve broke their allegiance to God by eating the forbidden fruit. Mankind's first sin would be a violation of a dietary command of God, a lack of self-control. Death and disease would now enter the world.

Man left Eden in sin and now must work the fields for his nourishment:

> **. . . and you will eat the plants of the field. (Genesis 3:18)**

In the early history of the Earth, man lived hundreds of years, or certainly longer than he lives today. He ate only fruits and vegetables and other vegetation. Because of the evil of man, God swept the Earth with the waters of the Great Flood. The vegetation was all destroyed, and the only immediate food source available to Noah and his family were the animals aboard the ark.

The food man would eat changed, and the life expectancy of man was appropriately shortened (perhaps to shorten man's sinful years). It is interesting to note the longevity change in man directly before and after the flood:

The life span of man ten generations before the flood.

| | | |
|---|---|---|
| Adam | 930 | years |
| Seth | 912 | |
| Enos | 905 | |
| Cainan | 910 | |
| Mahalaleel | 895 | |
| Jared | 962 | |
| Enoch | 365 | (translated) |
| Methuselah | 969 | |
| Lamech | 777 | |
| Noah | 950 | |
| | 912 | years average |

The life span of man ten generations after the flood.

| | | |
|---|---|---|
| Shem | 600 | (in childhood ate no meat) |
| Arphaxad | 438 | |
| Salah | 433 | |
| Eber | 464 | |
| Peleg | 239 | |
| Reu | 239 | |
| Serug | 230 | |
| Mahor | 148 | |
| Terah | 205 | |
| Abraham | 175 | |
| | 286 | years average (not including Shem) |

New directions regarding food selection were given:

> **Everything that lives and moves will be food for you. Just as I gave you the green plants, I now give you everything. (Genesis 9:3)**

Man could now eat anything that had once lived and moved, but God soon would be more specific as to exactly what could and could not be eaten in the animal world.

Thousands of years later, the value of God's original wish for man to enjoy the best of health by preferring a non-flesh diet was dramatically shown. The prophet Daniel was brought to Babylon by Nebuchadnezzar to learn the ways of his captor and to later enter the king's service. He was ordered to eat the royal food and drink, but Daniel would not eat in a way inconsistent with the requirements of God. Instead, he challenged his captors to prove their diet superior to his own:

> **"Please test your servants for ten days: Give us nothing but vegetables to eat and water to drink. Then compare our appearance with that of the young men who eat the royal food, and treat your servants in accordance with what you see." So he agreed to this and tested them for ten days. At the end of the ten days they looked healthier and better nourished than any of the young men who ate the royal food. So the guard took away their choice food and the wine they were to drink and gave them vegetables instead. (Daniel 1:12-16)**

**The Lord is good to all; he has compassion on all he has made. (Psalm 145:9)**

**How many are your works, O Lord! In wisdom you made them all; the earth is full of your creatures. (Psalm 104:24)**

## WE ARE ALL GOD'S CREATURES

One beautiful aspect of the Bible is that it provides us with a picture of God's ideal world. Knowing the ideal, we can assess our present status and develop goals for our constant improvement.

Were animals meant for food in God's original design for man in the idyllic Garden of Eden? When Eden is recreated in the New Earth, will man's relationship to the animal kingdom change?

In the Garden of Eden, Adam and Eve lived in perfect harmony with their environment and the animal kingdom. They derived their nutrition from plant life and not animal life. Only after the flood, when all vegetation was destroyed, were animals permitted to be used as food. However, harmony with the animal kingdom will again occur on earth:

**The wolf will live with the lamb,**
**the leopard will lie down with the goat,**
**the calf and the lion and the yearling together;**
**and a little child will lead them.**
**The cow will feed with the bear,**
**their young will lie down together,**
**and the lion will eat straw like the ox.**
**The infant will play near the hole of the cobra,**
**and the young child put his hand into the viper's nest.**
**They will neither harm nor destroy on all my holy mountain, for the earth will be full of the knowledge of the Lord as the waters cover the sea. (Isaiah 11:6-9)**

In the New Earth, life will be eternal for both man and animal. There will be no suffering. If there will be both no death and no suffering, then surely animals will not serve as food for man:

> **In that day I will make a covenant for them with the beasts of the field and the birds of the air and the creatures that move along the ground. Bow and sword and battle I will abolish from the land, so that all may lie down in safety. (Hosea 2:18)**

Does a God of kindness and mercy enjoy the slaughter of His animals in the name of food when better alternatives have been given to man?

We are again and again told to show kindness to all God's creatures. Unnecessary killing is not an act of kindness:

> **A righteous man cares for the needs of his animal, but the kindest acts of the wicked are cruel. (Proverbs 12:10)**

> **If you see the donkey of someone who hates you fallen down under its load, do not leave it there; be sure you help him with it. (Exodus 23:5)**

The fourth commandment of the precious Law of Moses regards the Sabbath day. Man, as well as animal, is to rest on this sacred day. It is a Sabbath for all God's creatures:

> **"Remember the Sabbath day by keeping it holy. Six days you shall labor and do all your work, but the seventh day is a Sabbath to the Lord your God. On it you shall not do any work, neither you, nor your son or daughter, nor your manservant or maidservant, nor your animals, nor the alien within your gates." (Exodus 20:8-10)**

**I will instruct you and teach you in the way you should go; I will counsel you and watch over you. Do not be like the horse or the mule, which have no understanding but must be controlled by bit and bridle or they will not come to you. Many are the woes of the wicked, but the Lord's unfailing love surrounds the man who trusts in him. (Psalm 32:8-10)**

## Second Nutritional Commandment
## THOU SHALL
## EAT ONLY "CLEAN" BIRDS, INSECTS, AND OTHER ANIMALS

After the time of the Great Flood, mankind was given very specific instructions regarding what life could be safely eaten. This nutritional guidance did not reflect the "trial and error" wisdom of early man, but was given by the Lord Himself to His spokesmen Moses and Aaron:

**" 'These are the regulations concerning animals, birds, every living thing that moves in the water and every creature that moves about on the ground. You must distinguish between the unclean and the clean, between living creatures that may be eaten and those that may not be eaten.' " (Leviticus 11:46,47)**

**" 'Of all the animals that walk on all fours, those that walk on their paws are unclean for you;' " (Leviticus 11:27)**

**These also shall be unclean unto you among the creeping things that creep upon the earth; the weasel, and the mouse, and the tortoise after his kind, and the ferret, and the chameleon, and the lizard, and the snail, and the mole. (Leviticus 11:29,30 KJV)**

**You may eat any clean bird. But these you may not eat: the eagle, the vulture, the black vulture, the red kite, the black kite, any kind of falcon, any kind of raven, the horned owl, the screech owl, the gull, any kind of hawk, the little owl, the great owl, the white owl, the desert owl, the osprey, the cormorant, the stork, any kind of heron, the hoopoe, and the bat. (Deuteronomy 14:11-18)**

**All flying insects that swarm are unclean to you; do not eat them. (Deuteronomy 14:19)**

**" 'All flying insects that walk on all fours are to be detestable to you. There are, however, some winged creatures that walk on all fours that you may eat: those that have jointed legs for hopping on the ground. Of these you may eat any kind of locust, katydid, cricket or grasshopper. But all other winged creatures that have four legs you are to detest.' " (Leviticus 11:20-23)**

**Do not eat anything you find already dead. (Deuteronomy 14:21)**

**Do not eat any detestable thing. These are the animals you may eat: the ox, the sheep, the goat, the deer, the gazelle, the roe deer, the wild goat, the ibex, the antelope and the mountain sheep. You may eat any animal that has a split hoof divided in two and that chews the cud. However, of those that chew the cud or that have a split hoof completely divided you may not eat the camel, the rabbit or the coney. Although they chew the cud, they do not have a split hoof; they are ceremonially unclean for you. (Deuteronomy 14:3-7)**

It is important that the reader know that a difference does exist between the different translations of the Bible, that this difference is at times significant, and usually reflects the personal religious bias of the interpreters more than an actual confusion within the original ancient Biblical manuscripts.

The Biblical version used for the purpose of this book is the New International Version (NIV), not necessarily for its literal translative accuracy, but for its contemporary simplicity in presentation. The King James Version (KJV), though Scripturally more original, is a bit distracting in its presentation, being written in an old English style.

The NIV states in Deuteronomy 14:7 that the above animals are *ceremonially* unclean, placing a unique meaning upon all of the previous text regarding those animals which should not be eaten by the faithful, observant people of God. In contrast, the KJV states, ". . . therefore they are unclean unto you." The word "ceremonially" is notably absent from the Scripture.

Should these animals be only ceremonially unclean, they would be permissable as food at that time when the ceremony was removed. Christ's original Apostles no longer observed tradition in connection with the eating of food. Yet, they still acknowledged and observed the distinction between clean and unclean animals, passed on to them from God and their forefathers (Acts 10:14, 2 Co. 6:17, 2 Co. 7:1). Apparently, these early Christians understood this passage in Deuteronomy to read, not like the NIV, but like the KJV.

It should be noted that the cow is a "clean" animal since its hoof is divided in two and it chews its cud. Its diet is that of an herbivore, seeking nourishment from no sources called "unclean" to man. The fat and blood of the cow, though, should be avoided as much as practically possible. The beef should be cooked well-done to remove all traces of blood or redness. Prolonged cooking will also help ensure the destruction of most potentially harmful micro-organisms within the beef.

Remember, healthy animals produce healthy meat. If one must eat meat, God encourages us to be selective in both our choice of the meat, and in its preparation.

**Be careful to follow every command I am giving you today, so that you may live and increase and may enter and possess the land that the Lord promised on oath to your forefathers. (Deuteronomy 8:1)**

## Third Nutritional Commandment
## THOU SHALL EAT ONLY FISH WITH FINS AND SCALES

All life requires food and all life produces waste. With that in mind, God has placed on earth two broad groups of animals; those which will act as food for man and those which will keep the earth clean by consuming man's wastes. In Biblical terms, those animals which are eatable to man are called "clean". The animals which sustain their own life by feeding off the waste products of man and other animals are termed "unclean". These scavenger animals were themselves never meant to be eaten by man, rather, their sole purpose is to provide a sanitary surrounding in which man can safely live.

Scavengers have been uniquely designed by God to ingest, without harm to themselves, that which is poisonous to man and other animals. To eat these unclean scavengers is to feast off the concentrated wastes of our environment:

**Of all the creatures living in the water of the seas and the streams, you may eat any that have fins and scales. (Leviticus 11:9)**

**Anything living in the water that does not have fins and scales is to be detestable to you. (Leviticus 11:12)**

**And since you are to detest them, you must not eat their meat and you must detest their carcasses. (Leviticus 11:11)**

Following is a list of the more commonly eaten forms of aquatic life. Discrimination has been made with respect to the presence of fins and scales, keeping in mind that in order for a fish to be suitable for eating it must have both present. There is slight disparity between modern zoological opinion and traditional religious views in developing this classification. However, any difference that does exist deals only with certain varieties within a particular fish family and this remains insignificant in light of the total picture.

| | *AQUATIC LIFE* | *FINS* | *SCALES* |
|---|---|---|---|
| | BASS | YES | YES |
| | BLUEFISH | YES | YES |
| | BLUEGILL | YES | YES |
| | BUFFALO | YES | YES |
| | CARP | YES | YES |
| * | CATFISH | YES | NO |
| * | CLAM | NO | NO |
| | COD | YES | YES |
| * | CRAB | NO | NO |
| * | EEL | NO | NO |
| | FLOUNDER | YES | YES |
| * | FROG | NO | NO |
| | HADDOCK | YES | YES |
| | HALIBUT | YES | YES |
| | HERRING | YES | YES |
| * | LOBSTER | NO | NO |
| | LOX | YES | YES |
| | MACKEREL | YES | YES |
| | MONKFISH | YES | YES |
| * | OCTOPUS | NO | NO |
| * | OYSTER | NO | NO |
| | PERCH | YES | YES |
| | POLLOCK | YES | YES |
| | POMPANO | YES | YES |
| | RAINBOW TROUT | YES | YES |
| | RED SNAPPER | YES | YES |
| | SALMON | YES | YES |
| * | SCALLOP | NO | NO |
| * | SHARK | YES | NO |
| * | SHRIMP | NO | NO |

| | *AQUATIC LIFE* | *FINS* | *SCALES* |
|---|---|---|---|
| | SMELT | YES | YES |
| | SOLE | YES | YES |
| * | SQUID | NO | NO |
| | STRIPED BASS | YES | YES |
| * | STURGEON | YES | NO |
| | SWORD FISH | YES | YES |
| | TUNA | YES | YES |
| | TURBOT | YES | YES |

* A FORBIDDEN FOOD FOR EITHER FINS OR SCALES ARE ABSENT

Concerning the proper conduct of the Christian, we read:

> **What does a believer have in common with an unbeliever? What agreement is there between the temple of God and idols? For we are the temple of the living God. As God has said: "I will live with them and walk among them, and I will be their God, and they will be my people." "Therefore come out from them and be separate, says the Lord. Touch no unclean thing, and I will receive you." (2 Corinthians 6:15-17)**

Paul's letter contains several important points key to our understanding of God's dietary commands:

1. The Christian is unique, having little in common with the non-believer, and should remain separate.
2. The Christian should abstain from eating, or even touching, unclean foods.
3. God will receive those who obey these commands.

Note the recognition of dietary guidelines by Paul in these writings in the New Testament. They are as relevant to the Christian church today as they were to the early Christian church of Corinth, to whom Paul directed this message.

**For even hereunto were ye called: because Christ also suffered for us, leaving us an example, that ye should follow his steps: (1 Peter 2:21 KJV)**

## WAS CHRIST A VEGETARIAN?

Adam and Eve lived in a land free of death, and the New Earth has been described as resembling Eden:

**Then I saw a new heaven and a new earth, for the first heaven and the first earth had passed away, and there was no longer any sea. (Revelation 21:1)**

**"He will wipe every tear from their eyes. There will be no more death or mourning or crying or pain, for the old order of things has passed away." (Revelation 21:4)**

Neither animal nor fish were slaughtered for food. The Earth's first inhabitants were vegetarian, and God's faithful followers that will later inherit the Earth will also be vegetarian.

Though Scripture strongly encourages the consumption of fruits and vegetables, proper obedience to the dietary laws does not demand abstinence from all meat and fish products. In Israel at the time of Jesus, meat and fish were commonly eaten. The faithful Israelite strictly followed the nutritional commandments of the Old Testament concerning "clean" and "unclean" foods. Later, the good Christians selectively choose their foods mindful of these same dietary laws.

Christ led His followers by both word and example. It was not His purpose to confuse early Christians, nor challenge the guidelines for proper Earthly existence set by His Father. For Christ to eat "clean" fish was neither sinful or contrary to sound Biblical doctrine.

Man has been pronounced, by God, as ruler over the animal kingdom. In God's covenant with Noah, man was told:

> **The fear and dread of you will fall upon all the beasts of the earth and all the birds of the air, upon every creature that moves along the ground, and upon all the fish of the sea; they are given into your hands. (Genesis 9:2)**

In like manner, the Psalmist describes man's dominion over fish and beast:

> **You made him ruler over the works of your hands; you put everything under his feet: all flocks and herds, and the beasts of the field, the birds of the air, and the fish of the sea, all that swim the paths of the seas. (Psalm 8:6-8)**

An early passage in Genesis lends further credence to the point:

> **Then God said, "Let us make man in our image, in our likeness, and let him rule over the fish of the sea and the birds of the air, over the livestock, over all the earth, and over all the creatures that move along the ground." (Genesis 1:26)**

In several passages, the eating of fish by Jesus is described. After the Resurrection, Jesus appeared to His disciples by the Sea of Galilee, who were fishing. Landing their boat ashore, the disciples saw a fire of burning coals with fish upon it. Bread was also there. (John 21:9) Jesus said to them:

> **"Come and have breakfast." None of the disciples dared ask him, "Who are you?" They knew it was the Lord. Jesus came, took the bread and gave it to them, and did the same with the fish. This was now the third time Jesus appeared to his disciples after he was raised from the dead. (John 21:12-14)**

In another instance following His death, Jesus offered to prove His real form to His disciples by having them touch His body:

> **Look at my hands and my feet. It is I myself! Touch me and see; a ghost does not have flesh and bones, as you see I have. (Luke 24:39)**

To show further proof of His genuineness, Christ offered to eat some food:

> **And while they still did not believe it because of joy and amazement, he asked them, "Do you have anything here to eat?" They gave him a piece of broiled fish, and he took it and ate it in their presence. (Luke 24:41-43)**

The commonly told story of Jesus feeding the multitudes with just a few fish and some bread, lends final evidence to Christ's dietary habits:

> **Taking the five loaves and the two fish and looking up to heaven, he gave thanks and broke the loaves. Then he gave them to his disciples to set before the people. He also divided the two fish among them all. They all ate and were satisfied, and the disciples picked up twelve basketfuls of broken pieces of bread and fish. The number of the men who had eaten was five thousand. (Mark 6:41-44)**

No evidence exists to support any premise that Christ ate meat or any "unclean" foods. But, Christ was not a vegetarian and neither must we be. If it be our aim to follow in Christ's footsteps, then we must draw a hard, discriminating line between those foods that are not Biblically allowed, and those which are sanctioned by God for our good health.

**He who scorns instruction will pay for it, but he who respects a command is rewarded. (Proverbs 13:13)**

## Fourth Nutritional Commandment
## THOU SHALL EAT NO BLOOD

As early as the Book of Genesis, God forbade Noah and his sons (of whom we all are) from eating meat with the blood of the animal still present:

> **"But you must not eat meat that has its lifeblood still in it." (Genesis 9:4)**

Similarly, the Lord told Moses to instruct the Israelites in like manner:

> **"And wherever you live, you must not eat the blood of any bird or animal." (Leviticus 7:26)**

We are to not only abstain from the ingestion of blood, but from the meat of strangled animals. Strangulation is a fairly slow form of death. Though animals were given by God to serve man, their torture is needless and should not be encouraged. Apostle James stated:

> **"Instead we should write to them, telling them to abstain from food polluted by idols, . . . from the meat of strangled animals and from blood." (Acts 15:20)**

The hunter, butcher, and chef all share a responsibility in ensuring that the animal is properly killed with minimal suffering and prepared as food with no trace of redness, or blood, in the meat:

> **But be sure you do not eat the blood, because the blood is the life, and you must not eat the life with the meat. You must not eat the blood; pour it out on the ground like water. Do not eat it, so that it may go well with you and your children after you, because you will be doing what is right in the eyes of the Lord. (Deuteronomy 12:23-25)**

The blood of man and animal serves two primary functions: a vehicle of transport for nutrients to the individual cells of the body, and a medium for the removal of waste products from those same cells. One can honestly define blood as unfiltered urine. To consume meat with the animal's blood still present is to consume the animal's waste products at the same time.

An antibody-antigen (allergic) (auto-immune) response occurs when we are exposed to human blood which is not of our own unique blood type. The pathologies associated with such an interaction progress on a continual scale from the relatively minor to allergy-induced shock and death. Perhaps this same type reaction occurs when we are exposed to the foreign proteins found within the blood of animals.

It is often for good, sound, scientific reason that God's nutritional and health message is appealing to us. But science is not always able to explain why we should behave in a certain manner. It is in these situations that we must rely upon our faith in a supreme being for direction. Therefore, like the Ten Commandments of Moses, we faithfully act because:

1. First, foremost, and of sufficient reason, we have a belief in God and we are told by Him to do so, and
2. Of no real importance, but satisfying to our mortal and erring minds, it may appeal to our present state of logic within the realm of science.

**See, I am setting before you today a blessing and a curse —the blessing if you obey the commands of the Lord your God that I am giving you today; the curse if you disobey the commands of the Lord your God and turn from the way that I command you today by following other gods, which you have not known. (Deuteronomy 11:26-28)**

## Fifth Nutritional Commandment
## THOU SHALL EAT NO FAT

Killing animals and using their meat for food is not encouraged by God among His people. Certain animals, if need be, can be used for food, but with their discriminate preparation. The blood and fat must be judiciously removed. It was not for unfounded reason that these directives were given, for today we see more clearly the wisdom of this advice:

**The Lord said to Moses, "Say to the Israelites: 'Do not eat any of the fat of cattle, sheep or goats. The fat of an animal found dead or torn by wild animals may be used for any other purpose, but you must not eat it.' " (Leviticus 7:22-24)**

This nation's present leading cause of death is heart disease. The issue of animal fat ingestion and its statistical relationship to coronary artery disease is well established. Fat ingestion is also strongly linked as a causative factor in cerebral stroke, diabetes mellitus, obesity, and certain forms of cancer. God, in His infinite wisdom, foresaw and recorded the nutritional cause of these various disorders well over two thousand years before science was able to provide a suitable explanation. Let us learn from this example. For the sake of brevity we must trust God, not science, for our nutritional advice.

**Be careful to obey all these regulations I am giving you, so that it may always go well with you and your children after you, because you will be doing what is good and right in the eyes of the Lord your God. (Deuteronomy 12:28)**

## Sixth Nutritional Commandment
## THOU SHALL EAT NO PORK

Early in man's history, God made known His desire concerning the ingestion of flesh from the pig:

**And the pig, though it has a split hoof completely divided, does not chew the cud; it is unclean for you. You must not eat their meat or touch their carcasses; they are unclean for you. (Leviticus 11:7,8)**

The eating of any unclean meat is a serious issue. It is undesirable from a health perspective, and a direct challenge to the wishes of our Master:

**All day long I have held out my hands to an obstinate people, who walk in ways not good, pursuing their own imaginations—a people who continually provoke me to my very face, . . . ; who eat the flesh of pigs, and whose pots hold broth of unclean meat; (Isaiah 65:2-4)**

Today, the pig is accepted as a source of food by many indiscriminate minds. It is eaten out of habit, while tastebuds sense enjoyment from this meat which society has learned to prepare in an appetizing way. The thought of eating a rat seems especially repulsive to these same individuals, though. Yet, rats and pigs are viewed in like manner by God, and neither should be eaten:

**"Those who consecrate and purify themselves to go into the gardens, following the one in the midst of those who eat the flesh of pigs and rats and other abominable things—they will meet their end together," declares the Lord. (Isaiah 66:17)**

Though God permitted the ingestion of meat by man since the time of the Great Flood, He was specific as to which meats would be least detrimental. Blood and fat are not to be eaten, for reasons more intricately explained by man much later in time. The meat of the pig, like other unclean meats, is also undesirable and is forbidden as food for God's people.

While it is indeed a poor decision from both Biblical and scientific perspectives to eat pork, we are also warned that even indirect contact with an unclean animal poses a threat to our health:

> **"Of all those that move along the ground, these are unclean for you. Whoever touches them when they are dead will be unclean till evening. When one of them dies and falls on something, that article, whatever its use, will be unclean, whether it is made of wood, cloth, hide or sackcloth. Put it in water; it will be unclean till evening, and then it will be clean. If one of them falls into a clay pot, everything in it will be unclean, and you must break the pot. Any food that could be eaten but has water on it from such a pot is unclean, and any liquid that could be drunk from it is unclean. Anything that one of their carcasses falls on becomes unclean; an oven or cooking pot must be broken up. They are unclean, and you are to regard them as unclean. A spring, however, or a cistern for collecting water remains clean, but anyone who touches one of these carcasses is unclean. If a carcass falls on any seeds that are to be planted, they remain clean. But if water has been put on the seed and a carcass falls on it, it is unclean for you. If an animal that you are allowed to eat dies, anyone who touches the carcass will be unclean till evening. Anyone who eats some of the carcass must wash his clothes, and he will be unclean till evening. Anyone who picks up the carcass must wash his clothes, and he will be unclean till evening." (Leviticus 11:31-40)**

For that temporary passing pleasure of a moment of culinary extravagance, we place both our physical and spiritual health in jeopardy. Can the logical mind in any way conclude that those hamhocks and pig's feet were in the final assessment, worth the price?

**Know also that wisdom is sweet to your soul; if you find it, there is future hope for you, and your hope will not be cut off. (Proverbs 24:14)**

## Seventh Nutritional Commandment
## THOU SHALL CONSUME NO ALCOHOL

The use of intoxicating beverages is an important health issue, and has rightfully been given much attention in the Bible. Alcoholic wine, and other fermented drinks, are responsible for the downfall of individuals and nations, priests and politicians, expectant mothers and seasoned warriors. It neither promotes physical vigor nor mental acquity. Its use is a shameful example of a personal lack of self-control, and certainly does not add to the glorification of God:

**Who has woe? Who has sorrow? Who has strife? Who has complaints? Who has needless bruises? Who has blood shot eyes? Those who linger over wine, who go to sample bowls of mixed wine. Do not gaze at wine when it is red, when it sparkles in the cup, when it goes down smoothly! In the end it bites like a snake and poisons like a viper. Your eyes will see strange sights and your mind imagine confusing things. You will be like one sleeping on the high seas, lying on top of the rigging. "They hit me," you will say, "but I'm not hurt! They beat me, but I don't feel it! When will I wake up so I can find another drink?" (Proverbs 23:29-35)**

In Paradise, Adam and Eve had access to fresh fruits and vegetables, and no directives were given by God to ferment these foods for drink. With the sin of man came death and disease. Only then do we read of the drinking of alcoholic wine and the evils associated with its consumption:

> **Noah, a man of the soil, proceeded to plant a vineyard. When he drank some of its wine, he became drunk and lay uncovered inside his tent. (Genesis 9:20,21)**

If our bodies are God's temples, is the drinking of alcohol, in any way, honoring our Maker? We are told:

> **Be self-controlled and alert, your enemy the devil prowls around like a roaring lion looking for someone to devour. (1 Peter 5:8)**

Far from enhancing our alertness, wine distorts our perception of reality and leads us further from God:

> **So then, let us not be like others, who are asleep, but let us be alert and self-controlled. For those who sleep, sleep at night, and those who get drunk, get drunk at night. But since we belong to the day, let us be self-controlled, putting on faith and love as a breast-plate, and the hope of salvation as a helmet. (1 Thessalonians 5:6-8)**

Drinkers of wine and doers of evil are alikened in the Bible:

> **In the hand of the Lord is a cup full of foaming wine mixed with spices; he pours it out, and all the wicked of the earth drink it down to its very dregs. (Psalm 75:8)**

According to Young's Analytical Concordance, the word "wine", in the context of the majority of the Bible, is defined as the juice pressed out from the grape, i.e. "grape juice". For example, we read:

> **Thus saith the Lord, As the new wine is found in the cluster, and one saith, Destroy it not; for a blessing is in it: so will I do for my servants' sakes, that I may not destroy them all. (Isaiah 65:8 KJV)**

With reference to this same Scripture, the New International Version states:

> **This is what the Lord says: "As when juice is still found in a cluster of grapes and men say, . . ."**

Theologians, apparently, do recognize the interchangeable nature of the words "wine" and "grape juice". In Scriptural discussions of drunkenness, though, wine is rightfully interpreted as an alcoholic drink. When in doubt concerning the meaning of the word "wine", one must interpret the word in light of the neighboring text and be mindful of the characters consuming the drink.

In the Book of John, chapter two, the story is told of Jesus changing water to wine. Contrary to the feelings of some misguided readers searching to justify their habit, this was not referring to alcoholic wine (fermented grape juice), but rather, to non-alcoholic wine (unfermented grape juice). It is illogical to assume that this wine was fermented, with reference to the over-all theme of the Bible's health message. It is also far-fetched to think that our Lord would encourage drunkenness among His followers by changing water to alcohol.

Jesus acted consistently with those principles revealed to earlier Biblical writers. In the Old Testament we read:

> **Wine is a mocker and beer a brawler; whoever is led astray by them is not wise. (Proverbs 20:1)**

In no instance in the Bible was Christ known to drink alcoholic wine. Note carefully what Christ did drink at the Last Supper:

> **Then he took the cup, gave thanks and offered it to them, saying, "Drink from it, all of you. This is my blood of the covenant, which is poured out for many for the forgiveness of sins. I tell you, I will not drink of this fruit of the vine from now on until that day when I drink it anew with you in my Father's kingdom." (Matthew 26:27-29)**

In Matthew 11:19, Christ was falsely accused of being a drunkard; the same false and degrading charges were made by others hoping to discredit the apostles (Acts 2:13), and Hannah (1 Samuel 1:12-16).

In another instance, Christ denied an offering of wine while walking to His Crucifixion:

> **Then they offered him wine mixed with myrrh, but he did not take it. (Mark 15:23)**

As our religious leaders must be of clear mind, so too must our nation's leaders not drink alcohol and so cloud their good judgement. Perhaps, we would be wise to judge the quality of potential political heads at election time by their personal habits as well as for their stand on various issues:

> **It is not for kings, O Lemuel—not for kings to drink wine, not for rulers to crave beer, lest they drink and forget what the law decrees, and deprive all the oppressed of their rights. (Proverbs 31:4,5)**
>
> **Then the Lord said to Aaron, "You and your sons are not to drink wine or other fermented drink whenever you go into the Tent of Meeting, or you will die." (Leviticus 10:8,9)**

Our God repeatedly gives man the opportunity to redeem himself from evil. But, if nations and individuals consistently choose to violate God's directives, this same free-will shall ultimately choose the path to their self-destruction:

> **This is what the Lord, the God of Israel, said to me: "Take from my hand this cup filled with the wine of my wrath and make all the nations to whom I send you drink it. When they drink it, they will stagger and go mad because of the sword I will send among them." (Jeremiah 25:15,16)**
>
> **"Then tell them, 'This is what the Lord Almighty, the God of Israel, says: Drink, get drunk and vomit, and fall to rise no more because of the sword I will send among you.' " (Jeremiah 25:27)**

No one is immune to the effects of alcohol, as priests and prophets are also warned to avoid its evils:

> **And these also stagger from wine and reel from beer: Priests and prophets stagger from beer and are befuddled with wine: they reel from beer, they stagger when seeing visions, they stumble when rendering decisions. (Isaiah 28:7)**

Directions are even given to the pregnant mother, God knowing that what she consumes during that important time, is also consumed by the unborn child:

**The angel of the Lord answered, "Your wife must do all that I have told her. She must not eat anything that comes from the grapevine, nor drink any wine or other fermented drink nor eat anything unclean. She must do everything I have commanded her." (Judges 13:13,14)**

Concerning the birth of John the Baptist, John's father Zechariah was told by an angel:

**He is never to take wine or other fermented drink, and he will be filled with the Holy Spirit even from birth. (Luke 1:15)**

The Bible presents a consistent argument against the use of alcoholic drinks. It warns of personal downfall:

**Do not get drunk on wine, which leads to debauchery. (Ephesians 5:18)**

It tells us not to associate with drunkards:

**. . . you must not associate with . . . a drunkard . . . (1 Corinthians 5:11)**

**Do not be misled: "Bad company corrupts good character." (1 Corinthians 15:33)**

The habit of drinking alcohol can only lead to harm. Let us learn from the history of others who have chosen a more sinful way:

**Their vine comes from the vine of Sodom and from the fields of Gomorrah. Their grapes are filled with poison, and their clusters with bitterness. Their wine is the venom of serpents, the deadly poison of cobras. (Deuteronomy 32:32,33)**

**Woe to those who rise early in the morning to run after their drinks, who stay up late at night till they are inflamed with wine. They have harps and lyres at their banquets, tambourines and flutes and wine, but they have no regard for the deeds of the Lord, no respect for the work of his hands. (Isaiah 5:11,12)**

**He who loves pleasure will become poor; whoever loves wine and oil will never be rich. (Proverbs 21:17)**

We are judged by both our faith and our actions. Earthly and heavenly punishment await those who choose not to follow the desires of God:

**"But as for you who forsake the Lord and forget my holy mountain, who spread a table for Fortune and fill bowls of mixed wine for Destiny, I will destine you for the sword, and you will bend down for the slaughter; for I called but you did not answer, I spoke but you did not listen. You did evil in my sight and chose what displeases me." (Isaiah 65:11,12)**

**Neither the . . . drunkards . . . will inherit the kingdom of God. (1 Corinthians 6:9,10)**

Like the Nazirites and the Recabites, and Jesus, we should seek heaven with a healthy body, clear mind, and respectful of all God's wishes. Unlike the Nazirites, though, it is not necessary to abstain from all grape products, unless that should be your own special vow of separation to the Lord:

**The Lord said to Moses, "Speak to the Israelites and say to them: 'If a man or woman wants to make a special vow, a vow of separation to the Lord as a Nazirite, he must abstain from wine and other fermented drink and must not drink vinegar made from wine or from other fermented drink. He must not drink grape juice or eat grapes or raisins. As long as he is a Nazirite, he must not eat anything that comes from the grapevine, not even the seeds or skins.' " (Numbers 6:1-4)**

**But they replied, "We do not drink wine, because our forefather Jonadab son of Recab gave us this command: 'Neither you nor your descendants must ever drink wine.' " (Jeremiah 35:6)**

**Be sober, be vigilant; because your adversary the devil, as a roaring lion, walketh about, seeking whom he may devour: (1 Peter 5:8 KJV)**

## SOBRIETY AND THE CHRISTIAN

Let there be no doubt; we are to confront reality with a sober mind and with righteous action. We are warned of an enemy searching among the prey of those whose defenses have been weakened by alcohol, whose minds are in a small way uncertain, whose memories are the least bit forgetful of God's plan for salvation. No mortal soul lies beyond the grasp of the devil. With even the clearest of minds and staunchest of characters, are we in any position to give Satan an advantage? We are reminded that even the pious bishop under the influence of alcohol will pose not a formidable foe to the supernatural powers of the devil. The hope of all men alone lies in clear, undistorted communication with Christ:

**This is a true saying, If a man desire the office of a bishop, he desireth a good work. A bishop then must be blameless, the husband of one wife, vigilant, sober, of good behaviour, given to hospitality, apt to teach; not given to wine, no striker, not greedy of filthy lucre; but patient, not a brawler, not covetous; (1 Timothy 3:1-3 KJV)**

Not just those of religious office are instructed to be of sober mind, but sobriety is a mark of obedience for all of God's people:

> **But speak thou the things which become sound doctrine: (Titus 2:1 KJV)**
>
> **That the aged men be sober, grave, temperate, sound in faith, in charity, in patience. (Titus 2:2 KJV)**
>
> **That they may teach the young women to be sober, to love their husbands, to love their children, (Titus 2:4 KJV)**
>
> **Young men likewise exhort to be sober minded. (Titus 2:6 KJV)**
>
> **For the grace of God that bringeth salvation hath appeared to all men, (Titus 2:11 KJV)**
>
> **Teaching us that, denying ungodliness and worldly lusts, we should live soberly, righteously, and godly, in this present world: (Titus 2:12 KJV)**

In a final warning, we are told:

> **Wherefore gird up the loins of your mind, be sober, and hope to the end for the grace that is to be brought unto you at the revelation of Jesus Christ; (1 Peter 1:13 KJV)**

**(Jesus replied to the Pharisees,)**
**"You have let go of the commands of God and are holding on to the traditions of men." (Mark 7:8)**

## Eighth Nutritional Commandment
## THOU SHALL EAT ONLY FOODS THAT HAVE ONCE HAD LIFE

Biblical man was not concerned with the dangers of food additives, preservatives, artificial colorings, highly processed foods, refined foods, and food substitutes. God in His eternal wisdom, though, foresaw the day when man would choose not to eat foods in the manner that he had provided.

The Master Designer of our body knows best what foods should be sought for our nourishment. If God wanted our cheese to be processed, milk to be homogenized and sugar to be refined, is it not logical to think that our Creator would have provided these foods in that form originally? If our fruits are in need of coloring or our vegetables in need of flavoring, let nature provide that extra ingredient. God's gifts to us would do well without man's chemical adulteration:

**Everything that lives and moves will be food for you. Just as I gave you the green plants, I now give you everything. (Genesis 9:3)**

We are given two criteria in choosing food:

1. It must have lived, and
2. It must have moved.

Genesis 9:3 does not mean that all life is edible, for many exclusions had later been placed upon this generalized category. The category is specific, though, to the plant and animal kingdom. Certainly, animals both live and move and plants move by growing, but additives, preservatives, and synthetic foods present themselves as laboratory concoctions and meet neither of these criteria.

God has said that if we violate His commands we will be struck with "wasting diseases" (Deuteronomy 28:22). Cancer is a wasting disease. But has a banana or an apple or a pear ever been associated with this disease? However, many food-colorings and additives have been labeled as cancer causing agents and should wisely be avoided.

Relying upon science for his direction, mankind is often mislead. We are reminded in Proverbs that the animal kingdom has not been so delusioned and continues to seek its food in an intelligent way:

> **Go to the ant, you sluggard; consider its ways and be wise! It has no commander, no overseer or ruler, yet it stores its provisions in summer and gathers its food at harvest. (Proverbs 6:6-8)**

We should also consider Leviticus 25:7, though, which is not an open invitation to eat *anything* the land produces. Common sense leads us away from eating oak trees and thorn bushes. We *are* told, however, to look at what God pushes up through the soil as food for our nourishment:

> **Whatever the land produces may be eaten. (Leviticus 25:7)**

Acts 14:17 is quite a beautiful Scripture. In all of nature is evidence of God's presence. We would be wise to accept God's gifts to us, unchanged and in their original form:

> **"Yet he has not left himself without testimony: He has shown kindness by giving you rain from heaven and crops in their seasons; he provides you with plenty of food and fills your hearts with joy." (Acts 14:17)**

> **Finally, brothers, good-by. Aim for perfection, listen to my appeal, be of one mind, live in peace. And the God of love and peace will be with you. (2 Corinthians 13:11)**

## MILK AND CHEESE (IN ITS ORIGINAL FORM)

Though not a part of the early dietary practices of Adam and Eve, the use of milk and cheese became a regular part of the eating style of the early Biblical people:

> **Then he (Abraham) ran to the herd and selected a choice, tender calf and gave it to a servant, who hurried to prepare it. He then brought come curds and milk and the calf that had been prepared, and set these before them. While they ate, he stood near them under a tree. (Genesis 18:7,8)**

> **". . . a land flowing with milk and honey . . ." (Exodus 3:8)**

> **He nourished him with honey from the rock, and with oil from the flinty crag, with curds and milk from herd and flock . . . (Deuteronomy 32:13,14)**

> **"I'm thirsty," he said. "Please give me some water." She opened a skin of milk, gave him a drink, and covered him up. (Judges 4:19)**

> **You will have plenty of goats' milk to feed you and your family and to nourish your servant girls. (Proverbs 27:27)**

> **therefore I am going to give you to the people of the East as a possession. They will set up their camps and pitch their tents among you; they will eat your fruit and drink your milk. (Ezekiel 25:4)**

With milk becoming a customary part of the diet, it is to be expected that cheese should also become a commonly eaten food:

> **They also brought wheat and barley, flour and roasted grains, beans and lentils, honey, curds and sheep, and cheese from cows' milk for David and his people to eat. For they said, "The people have become hungry and tired and thirsty in the desert." (2 Samuel 17:28,29)**
>
> **Now Jesse said to his son David, "Take this ephah of roasted grain and take these ten loaves of bread for your brothers and hurry to their camp. Take along these ten cheeses to the commander of their unit. See how your brothers are and bring back some assurance from them." (1 Samuel 17:17,18)**

From a health perspective, we must remember that milk can be no healthier than the animal from which it comes, and that the adulteration of milk through present-day processing methods makes it a food quite unlike its original form.

**No temptation has seized you except what is common to man. And God is faithful; he will not let you be tempted beyond what you can bear. But when you are tempted, he will also provide a way out so that you can stand up under it. (1 Corinthians 10:13)**

## Ninth Nutritional Commandment
## THOU SHALL SHOW MODERATION WHEN EATING

**You must teach what is in accord with sound doctrine. Teach the older men to be temperate, worthy of respect, self-controlled, and sound in faith, in love and endurance. (Titus 2:1,2)**

**Similarly, encourage the young men to be self-controlled. (Titus 2:6)**

**Like a city whose walls are broken down is a man who lacks self-control. (Proverbs 25:28)**

The subject of proper nutrition extends beyond the discriminate selection of foods, but includes the topic of moderation in the ingestion of the right foods. It is only marginally better to be overweight from eating carrots than from eating pork, for body fat is identical regardless of its original source. We all do possess self-control, though, if we should so choose to use it. It is an outward sign of our choosing to follow God:

**For the grace of God that brings salvation has appeared to all men. It teaches us to say "No" to ungodliness and worldly passions, and to live self-controlled, upright and godly lives in this present age. (Titus 2:11,12)**

Moderation when eating is a small sacrifice in comparison to Christ's greater sacrifice for us:

> **Therefore, since Christ suffered in his body, arm yourselves also with the same attitude, because he who has suffered in his body is done with sin. As a result, he does not live the rest of his earthly life for evil human desires, but rather for the will of God. For you have spent enough time in the past doing what pagans choose to do —living in debauchery, lust, drunkenness, orgies, carousing and detestable idolatry. (1 Peter 4:1-3)**

The issue of moderate intake pertains to all foods:

> **Eat honey, my son, for it is good; honey from the comb is sweet to your taste. (Proverbs 24:13)**

> **If you find honey, eat just enough—too much of it, and you will vomit. (Proverbs 25:16)**

The rules of God pertain to all men. Food at proper times is refreshing and necessary; in excess, leads to ill health:

> **Blessed are you, O land whose king is of noble birth and whose princes eat at a proper time—for strength and not for drunkenness. (Ecclesiastes 10:17)**

God has stated what is proper. Satan provokes the sin of man by tempting us with the improper by appealing to our lusts:

> **When you sit to dine with a ruler, note well what is before you, and put a knife to your throat if you are given to gluttony. Do not crave his delicacies, for that food is deceptive. (Proverbs 23:1-3)**

The Great Commandment, "Thou Shall Not Kill," can be directed in purpose not only to the killing of one's fellow man, but also to the destruction of one's self through the insidious route of ill-health:

> **Do not join those who drink too much wine or gorge themselves on meat, for drunkards and gluttons become poor, and drowsiness clothes them in rags. (Proverbs 23:20,21)**

Jeshurun showed contempt for God not only in his attitude, but in his actions which lacked self-denial:

> **Jeshurun grew fat and kicked; filled with food, he became heavy and sleek. He abandoned the God who made him and rejected the Rock his Savior. (Deuteronomy 32:15)**

The inter-relationship of attitude and proper action is simply and distinctly stated in Paul's message to the Galatians:

> **But the fruit of the Spirit is love, joy, peace, patience, kindness, goodness, faithfulness, gentleness and self-control. (Galatians 5:22,23)**

The relationship between gluttony, lack of self-control, obesity, and overweight, is obvious. Overweight is a relative term, and there is some degree of damage to the body each step along the continuim. The effects of carrying excessive poundage are mainly cardiovascular, but truly influence every part of the body in some way. It is not difficult to imagine every system in the body working harder to deal with the stress of the unnecessary weight. The heart beats harder, the lungs breathe laboriously, the muscles strain, and the skeleton is burdened. The quality of life is affected. God is not honored when the body is abused, as one's lust for food becomes master over reason.

Ample evidence is present to encourage the rational mind and the obedient Christian to show self-control with regard to the ingestion of food. Knowledge without action is of little value. Let us put what we know to be right into effect.

> **For, as I have often told you before and now say again even with tears, many live as enemies of the cross of Christ. Their destiny is destruction, their god is their stomach, and their glory is in their shame. (Philippians 3:18,19)**

**"Even now," declares the Lord, "return to me with all your heart, with fasting and weeping and mourning." (Joel 2:12)**

## Tenth Nutritional Commandment
## THOU SHALL FAST IN TIMES OF NEED

While the intelligent selection of food is essential to maintaining good health, conscious and proper abstinence from food is, at times, crucial to health's restoration. Disorders from the excesses of food are obviously, adequately managed by selective dieting. As God has provided for us a plan for all of life's situations, so too has a plan been revealed for the care of those times of ill-health. Food, again, is a key. Simply, we must know when to eat, and when not to eat if we want to enjoy the good health that God desires us to have.

To not eat food is to fast; Christ tells us so in the accounts of Matthew 15:32 (KJV) and Mark 8:2,3 (KJV):

**Then Jesus called his disciples unto him, and said, I have compassion on the multitude, because they continue with me now three days, and have nothing to eat: I will not send them away fasting, lest they faint in the way. (Matthew 15:32 KJV)**

Biblical history is replete with key figures who practiced the art of fasting. Our list includes such noteables as:

| | |
|---|---|
| Moses (Exodus 34:27,28) | Samuel (1 Samuel 7:5,6) |
| Israelites (Judges 20:26) | David (2 Samuel 12:16) |
| Elijah (1 Kings 19:8) | Ninevites (Jonah 3:5-8) |
| Nehemiah (Nehemiah 1:4) | Darius (Daniel 6:9,18) |
| Daniel (Daniel 9:3) | Anna (Luke 2:36,37) |
| Jesus (Matthew 4:1,2) | Paul (2 Corinthians 11:27) |
| Early Christians (Acts 13:2) | Apostles (2 Corinthians 6:4,5) |

John's disciples and the Pharisees (Mark 2:18)

For good reason did such a noteworthy group choose to periodically abstain from food. Our Biblical friends were motivated by unfulfilled needs similar to those found in present society:

**Need for Divine Guidance.** Some situations are far too difficult to comprehend, with variables too numerous to master. In Judges 20:26-28 we are given the following account of the Israelites communicating with God, seeking clarity of mind through fasting:

> **Then the Israelites, all the people, went up to Bethel, and there they sat weeping before the Lord. They fasted that day until evening and presented burnt offerings and fellowship offerings to the Lord. And the Israelites inquired of the Lord. (In those days the ark of the covenant of God was there, with Phinehas son of Eleazar, the son of Aaron, ministering before it.) They asked, "Shall we go up again to battle with Benjamin our brother, or not?" The Lord responded, "Go, for tomorrow I will give them into your hands." (Judges 20:26-28)**

**Need for Victory Over Temptation.** Paul tells us that there is strength to be gotten in times of weakness:

> **That is why, for Christ's sake, I delight in weakness, in insults, in hardships, in persecutions, in difficulties. For when I am weak, then I am strong. (2 Corinthians 12:10)**

The account of Christ's battle and victory with the Great Tempter presents to us an example of the character building value of fasting:

> **Then Jesus was led by the Spirit into the desert to be tempted by the devil. After fasting forty days and forty nights, he was hungry. The tempter came to him and said, "If you are the Son of God, tell these stones to become bread." Jesus answered, "It is written: 'Man does not live on bread alone, but on every word that comes from the mouth of God.' " (Matthew 4:1-4)**

**Need for Victory Over Ill-Health.** There is a wholeness of man, an inter-relationship of Spirit, Mind, and Body. That affecting one part affects the other sides of this triad. While fasting favorably affects the spiritual and psychological aspects of man, Scripture also notes a positive influence upon the physical side. The Book of Isaiah concludes its discussion of fasting with the following, firmly encouraging the practice of fasting for physical health:

> **Then your light will break forth like the dawn, and your healing will quickly appear; then your righteousness will go before you, and the glory of the Lord will be your rear guard. (Isaiah 58:8)**

Health is again related to fasting in the account of Jesus and the epileptic:

> **And Jesus rebuked the devil; and he departed out of him: and the child was cured from that very hour. Then came the disciples to Jesus apart, and said, Why could not we cast him out? And Jesus said unto them, Because of your unbelief: for verily I say unto you, If ye have faith as a grain of mustard seed, ye shall say unto this mountain, Remove hence to yonder place; and it shall remove; and nothing shall be impossible unto you. Howbeit this kind goeth not out but by prayer and fasting. (Matthew 17:18-21 KJV)**

Interestingly, and of no minor note, we are told by Jesus that fasting is expected from His faithful followers:

> **Then John's disciples came and asked him, "How is it that we and the Pharisees fast, but your disciples do not fast?" Jesus answsered, "How can the guests of the bridegroom mourn while he is with them? The time will come when the bridegroom will be taken from them; then they *will* fast." (Matthew 9:14,15)**

Fasting, though, is more than just abstaining from food. We are told that it is to be done in humbleness, as we chasten our soul in prayer:

> **Yet when they were ill, I put on sackcloth and humbled myself with fasting. (Psalm 35:13)**
>
> **When I wept, and chastened my soul with fasting, that was to my reproach. (Psalm 69:10 KJV)**
>
> **So I turned to the Lord God and pleaded with him in prayer and petition, in fasting, and in sackcloth and ashes. (Daniel 9:3)**

Finally, fast not as a spectacle, but in the privacy of a relationship between oneself and God:

> **"When you fast, do not look somber as the hypocrites do, for they disfigure their faces to show men they are fasting. I tell you the truth, they have received their reward in full. But when you fast, put oil on your head and wash your face, so that it will not be obvious to men that you are fasting, but only to your Father, who is unseen; and your Father, who sees what is done in secret, will reward you." (Matthew 6:16-18)**

When contemplating our own Christian sacrifice, let us remember well the lifestyle of the faithful Apostle Paul:

> **In weariness and painfulness, in watchings often, in hunger and thirst, in fastings often, in cold and nakedness. (2 Corinthians 11:27 KJV)**

We are all in need of uplifting human examples upon whom we can pattern at least a portion of our own life. The Bible provides us with the highpoints of the outstanding people of history. What simpler way to personal success than to mimic those who have already achieved their share of greatness. "In fasting often," we too can enjoy a common bond with our forcfathers of the Bible, and meet well those special needs.

**And as for you, brothers, never tire of doing what is right. (2 Thessalonians 3:13)**

**Endure hardship as discipline; God is treating you as sons. (Hebrews 12:7)**

## STRIVE FOR PHYSICAL PERFECTION

Our usefulness as a worker for God depends upon our good health. Constantly work toward its perfection, and seek ways of bettering all that you do. Make that extra effort to select the choicest apple, to grow the finest crop, to improve the combination of foods in your diet. Expand your knowledge of the plant kingdom. Study better ways of preparing meals, of making that salad more nutritious, of cooking those vegetables more efficiently. Raise the quality of all that you eat, to in turn, raise the quality of your own good health:

**Don't you know that you yourselves are God's temple and that God's Spirit lives in you? If anyone destroys God's temple, God will destroy him; for God's temple is sacred, and you are that temple. (1 Corinthians 3:16,17)**

**Do you not know that your body is a temple of the Holy Spirit, who is in you, whom you have received from God? You are not your own; you were bought at a price. Therefore honor God with your body. (1 Corinthians 6:19,20)**

Do you not know that your bodies are members of Christ himself? (1 Corinthians 6:15)

Therefore, I urge you, brothers, in view of God's mercy, to offer your bodies as living sacrifices, holy and pleasing to God—which is your spiritual worship. (Romans 12:1)

Be perfect, therefore, as your heavenly Father is perfect. (Matthew 5:48)

Since we have these promises, dear friends, let us purify ourselves from everything that contaminates body and spirit, perfecting holiness out of reverence for God. (2 Corinthians 7:1)

For this is the reason the gospel was preached even to those who are now dead, so that they might be judged according to men in regard to the body, but live according to God in regard to the spirit. (1 Peter 4:6)

Still others, like seed sown among thorns, hear the word; but the worries of this life, the deceitfulness of wealth and the desires for other things come in and choke the word, making it unfruitful. (Mark 4:18)

Whoever gives heed to instruction prospers, and blessed is he who trusts in the Lord. (Proverbs 16:20)

**The mocker seeks wisdom and finds none, but knowledge comes easily to the discerning. (Proverbs 14:6)**

## IN RESPONSE TO THE NON-BELIEVERS

In preparing this work, I soon realized that certain Scriptures exist and that certain viewpoints prevail which draw confusion to the basic theme of this book.

The word "health" is a relative word. One can always be healthier regardless of his present state of being. Ideally, we should strive for the original state of man, as found in the Garden of Eden.

Adam and Eve consumed a diet of mostly fruits and some vegetables. One would suspect that all the food was raw. There was no mention of prepared foods, the eating of animals or animal products such as milk, large sit-down meals, or fermented beverages. The food was fresh, unadulterated, and of plant origin.

With Adam in mind, these Ten Nutritional Commandments should be critically evaluated. The eating of certain meats is now allowed, ideally though, no meat should be consumed. Certain fish are also now permissable, but again, Adam in his idyllic state did not eat fish. The need to discriminate between "clean" birds, insects, and other animals was of no concern in Eden, for no animal life, "clean" or "unclean", was eaten. In our striving for physical perfection we must remember first the ideal, secondly, the permissable, and finally, that which under no conditions is allowable.

> **They forbid people to marry and order them to abstain from certain foods, which God created to be received with thanksgiving by those who believe and who know the truth. For everything God created is good, and nothing is to be rejected if it is received with thanksgiving, because it is consecrated by the word of God and prayer. (1 Timothy 4:3-5)**

All that God created *is* good; but not all that God created is good for food. The thought of eating all of God's creations is illogical, and not in line with the overwhelming theme of the Bible. All that God created has a purpose. That which was created as food for man has been so labeled in earlier passages of the Bible, and that which is not to be eaten has also been appropriately marked.

The warning is well made to beware of those who forbid people to marry and abstain from certain foods. Marriage is the basis of the Christian home and is encouraged, not discouraged, in Scripture. We also need not abstain from any food which has been labeled as food, but we are to abstain from that which is eatable yet has been labeled as "unclean", and is therefore not a food. That which God created as food for our nourishment is meant for our useful consumption and to be received, like all that God has given us, with thanksgiving.

Each and every word in Scripture is carefully placed, and meaningful. In one's haste, a person may casually read a passage and misinterpret its proper meaning. The Gospel of Matthew provides us with a good example of this:

> **Then some Pharisees and teachers of the law came to Jesus from Jerusalem and asked, "Why do your disciples break the tradition of the elders? They don't wash their hands before they eat!" (Matthew 15:1,2)**

This was a ritualistic washing, and not a sanitary one. A small amount of water was poured on the fingers and a little on the hand, not enough for cleansing but enough to satisfy the ancient tradition.

Christ replied to the Pharisees:

> **"Don't you see that whatever enters the mouth goes into the stomach and then out of the body? But the things that come out of the mouth come from the heart, and these make a man 'unclean.' " (Matthew 15:17,18)**

Some have used this passage of Scripture as an excuse to ignore God's health laws, and therefore, partake of all manner of "unclean" foods. However, when this passage is examined in its context and the true meaning is discovered, it becomes quite clear that it is not referring to food at all. Christ was responding to the question posed by the Pharisees which inferred that those who do not wash their hands before eating are made "unclean" by such action. Christ denied the validity of the Pharisees' interpretation of this tradition. Contrary to their opinion, improperly washed hands, from a ritualistic standpoint, do not cause defilement of the individual. The thought, and the expression of the thought verbally and by action, is what makes a man "unclean".

Certain Scriptures, when viewed out of context, have the potential of being misleading to the reader. The Book of Acts discusses a dream that Peter had upon a rooftop. He saw Heaven open and all kinds of animals appear:

> **Then a voice told him, "Get up, Peter. Kill and eat."**
> **"Surely not, Lord!" Peter replied. "I have never eaten anything impure or unclean."**
> **The voice spoke to him a second time, "Do not call anything impure that God has made clean."**
> **This happened three times, and immediately the sheet was taken back to heaven. (Acts 10:13-16)**

Of note is the fact that Peter, one of the original twelve apostles of Christ, should still practice dietary restrictions, even after Christ's death. Some, however, believe that this statement is saying that one should not continue such self-denial, that there is no difference between "clean" and "unclean" animals.

Reading further, Peter's interpretation of the dream is revealed:

> **He said to them: "You are well aware that it is against our law for a Jew to associate with a Gentile or visit him. But God has shown me that I should not call any man impure or unclean. (Acts 10:28)**

Peter's vision was not concerned with food at all! The "clean" and "unclean" animals envisioned were used symbolically to represent the mingling of Jews and Gentiles, a practice which had earlier been discouraged.

Another potentially misleading Scripture is found in Colossians:

> **Therefore do not let anyone judge you by what you eat or drink, or with regard to a religious festival, a New Moon celebration or a Sabbath Day. These are a shadow of the things that were to come; the reality, however, is found in Christ. (Colossians 2:16,17)**

This does not mean, as some think, that one can now eat or drink anything. Mankind has not physically changed to a significant enough degree to now allow the healthy consumption of any food or drink. Nor has God made any statement that man can now eat anything, irrespective of His earlier directives, or that food has no relation to physical health. This is obviously incorrect. Colossians 2:16 does tell us, though, not to *judge* our fellow man by what they eat or drink. Judgement is not our duty, but is solely the duty of our Creator:

> **"Do not judge, or you too will be judged." (Matthew 7:1)**

However, while we should not judge another, we should remember that one day we will be judged against the things that are written in the Bible, health principles included.

The Apostle Paul has authored many of the writings of the New Testament. Several of his statements may lead the reader to believe that he felt, with the death of Christ, the Christian was removed of all obligation to the prior commandments of God and all the laws of Moses. Paul, however, expressed his faithfulness to these earlier directives at his trial with Festus. Being accused of teaching the Jews to turn away from Moses and to not live according to their customs (Acts 21:21), Paul responded:

> **"I have done nothing wrong against the law of the Jews or against the temple or against Caesar." (Acts 25:8)**

In his trial before Felix for similar charges, Paul replied in a similar manner:

> **"However, I admit that I worship the God of our fathers, as a follower of the Way, which they call a sect. I believe everything that agrees with the Law and that is written in the Prophets, . . . (Acts 24:14)**

Should confusion arise concerning the meaning of an unclear passage, it would be wise to consider the context in which it was written, the customs prevalent at that time, the persuasion of the writer, and paralleling Scriptures:

> **Above all, you must understand that no prophecy of Scriptures came about by the prophet's own interpretation. For prophecy never had its origin in the will of man, but men spoke from God as they were carried along by the Holy Spirit. (2 Peter 1:20,21)**

In a situation similar to Paul's, the Apostle Stephen was falsely accused of preaching that Jews and Christians no longer need adhere to God's commandments as found in the Old Testament. Unable to argue effectively against Stephen, the members of the Synagogue brought false testimony against the apostle:

> **Then they secretly persuaded some men to say, "We have heard Stephen speak words of blasphemy against Moses and against God." So they stirred up the people and the elders and the teachers of the law. They seized Stephen and brought him before the Sanhedrin. They produced false witnesses, who testified, "This fellow never stops speaking against the holy place and against the law. For we have heard him say that this Jesus of Nazareth will destroy this place and change the customs Moses handed down to us." (Acts 6:11-14)**

If this is an honest description of what the false accusers said regarding the teachings of Stephen, then the opposite must be true. Stephen, like Paul and Peter, upheld the ancient commandments of God, realizing that these laws had not changed with the coming of Christ.

In a discussion of the weak and strong of faith, Romans includes the following statements regarding diet:

> **One man's faith allows him to eat everything, but another man, whose faith is weak, eats only vegetables. (Romans 14:2)**
>
> **As one who is in the Lord Jesus, I am fully convinced that no food is unclean in itself. But if anyone regards something as unclean, then for him it is unclean. (Romans 14:14)**

The total passage is summarized with two statements identified by the key word, "therefore."

> **Therefore let us stop passing judgment on one another. Instead, make up your mind not to put any stumbling block or obstacle in your brother's way. (Romans 14:13)**
>
> **Let us therefore make every effort to do what leads to peace and to mutual edification. Do not destroy the work of God for the sake of food. All food is clean, but it is wrong for a man to eat anything that causes someone else to stumble. (Romans 14:19,20)**

These statements by Paul parallel a similar passage (Colossians 2:16) previously discussed regarding judgment of your fellow man. The general theme of these writings is not that of disrupting the health/dietary guidelines that have stood since man's conception, but of encouraging harmony between Christians with varying degrees of conviction. Remember, swine and other "unclean" meats are not considered food by the Jews and early Christians. All food is "clean", but if someone decides that he personally will not eat some of the "clean" food, then for him that food should not be eaten and may be called "unclean" in that person's eye. The Nazarites, for example, would not eat grapes or raisins, though they are "clean" and permissable foods. For the Nazarite, the raisin is "unclean" and should not be eaten (Numbers 6:1-4). Their unique practice should not be considered a rule for all Christians, and should likewise not be a center of controversy among those striving to be faithful.

**This is what the Lord says: "Cursed is the one who trusts in man, who depends on flesh for his strength and whose heart turns away from the Lord." (Jeremiah 17:5)**

**"But blessed is the man who trusts in the Lord, whose confidence is in him." (Jeremiah 17:7)**

## RELY ON GOD FOR YOUR HEALTH

Good health is not a simplistic issue. Exercise, psychological stability, rest, fresh air, spiritual fulfillment and other important factors must be considered. Proper nutrition is also essential and it is that issue which is addressed in this book.

Our Maker desires to see His creations enjoy good health, and He has presented rules for meeting this objective. Man's free will allows him to disobey God by not following His nutritional laws and thus not enjoying the best of health, or being faithful subjects willing to submit to our Creator's directives, and harvesting the physical rewards of vitality and lessened chance of disease.

Summarizing the previous text, God strictly forbids certain foods from our diet, encourages the consumption of other foods, and allows selection within another group of less desirable foodstuffs.

In line with God's wishes, we would do well to follow His nutritional guidelines. We are told to:

1. Prefer fruits, vegetables, nuts, grains, and seeds.
2. Avoid the ingestion of all animal meats and animal products.
3. Strictly avoid eating pork and the meat of all other "unclean" animals.
4. Eat only the meat of "clean" animals. As much fat should be stripped away as practically possible, and the meat prepared well to remove all traces of blood or redness.
5. Completely avoid the consumption of alcohol.
6. Avoid man-made foods and artificial food ingredients.
7. Eat in moderation, and only to satisfy your hunger.
8. Seek variety in one's selection of foods from the plant kingdom.
9. Prepare food with minimal alteration to the original state of the product.
10. Fast often for spiritual, psychological, and physical well-being.

**Do not merely listen to the word, and so deceive yourselves. Do what it says. (James 1:22)**

**Now all has been heard; here is the conclusion of the matter: Fear God and keep his commandments, for this is the whole duty of man. (Ecclesiastes 12:13)**

# A SCRIPTURAL INDEX

## Old Testament

**New Testament**